The Fatty Liver Diet and Cookbook

Beat Fatty Liver with Diet and Lifestyle Changes

Kenneth Martin

Acknowledgement

Getting a book written, proofed and published is no small job. I want to thank the many people that were instrumental in bringing this idea to life. In particular, I would like to thank friends and family for helping me with the selection, editing and proofreading of this book.

Table of Contents

Introduction

The Fatty Liver Diet and Cookbook, was written for those who currently may have a Fatty Liver Condition as an easy-to-use tool for understanding and either reversing it or avoiding it altogether.

Its concise and practical approach is meant to provide a framework for understanding just what Fatty Liver Disease is all about.

In recent years, there's been an explosion of Fatty Liver Disease. Simply put, the more obese we become as a nation, the more instances of it. Arguably, this rise is being driven by our increasing sedentary lifestyles coupled with our intake of processed food.

Fatty Liver disease develops over time and we are normally indirectly or directly are the culprit for its development. It is the build-up of extra fat in the liver cells. If more than 5% to 10% of the liver's weight is fatty, then it is called fatty liver—steatosis. On the other hand, should your liver become inflamed, this is called steatohepatitis. Once there is a build-up of fat the liver does becomes vulnerable to inflammation and scarring.

Fatty liver disease tends to develop in people who are overweight or obese or have diabetes, high cholesterol or high triglycerides/ lipids. This is a result of defective fatty acid metabolism and is normally caused by poor eating habits, too much alcohol or even certain medications.

In any event, left unchecked Fatty Liver Disease can lead to Cirrosis of the liver which could ultimately be deadly.

The good news, however, is that condition is reversible and that the liver is a very resilient organ. You should ensure that you follow these simple rules of thumb to either avoid it or ward it off:

- Limit alcoholic beverages and drinks sweetened with fruit sugar (fructose). Instead, drink plenty of nonalcoholic beverages, especially water.

- Exercise regularly and lose weight. Keeping your body at a healthy weight reduces your risk of Fatty Liver Disease.

- Limit sugary products such as candy and desserts that tend to be high in calories that tend to lead to obesity.

Having said that, this doesn't mean that your taste buds have to be affected. In the first part of this book we put into perspective just what Fatty Liver is. In the latter part of the book we present a vast array of friendly food and meal options that covers everything from Breakfast to Dessert.

Eat up & enjoy.

Chapter 1: What is the Liver?

We can't live without a functioning liver!

Almost all cells and tissues in the body depend upon the liver. The liver serves as the body's filter and warehouse. A little over 1 ½ quarts of blood pump through the liver every minute, allowing it to quickly and effectively remove toxins and waste products from the blood stream. It also acts as a warehouse to hold onto substances like vitamins, minerals and glucose that the body will need later. The liver helps to manage cholesterol, hormones and sugar. It regulates fat storage and blood clotting factors.

What does my liver look like?

The liver is the largest organ inside the body. In an adult, it is about the size of a football and weighs close to three pounds. It is located behind the ribs in the upper right-hand portion of the abdomen. Shaped like a triangle, the liver is dark reddish-brown and consists of two main lobes. There are over 300 billion specialized cells in the liver that are connected by a well organized system of bile ducts and blood vessels called the biliary system.

How important is my liver?

The liver is such an important organ that we can survive only one or two days if it shuts down—if the liver fails, your body will fail, too. Fortunately, the liver can function even when up to 75% of it is diseased or removed. This is because it has the amazing ability to create new liver tissue regenerate its from healthy liver cells that still exist.

What does my liver do?

The liver does hundreds of vital things to make sure everything runs smoothly. That said, some of the most important functions of the liver include:

- Stores vitamins, sugar and iron to help give your body energy.
- Controls the production and removal of cholesterol.
- Clears your blood of waste products, drugs, and other poisonous substances.
- Makes clotting factors to stop excessive bleeding after cuts or injuries.
- Produces immune factors and removes bacteria from the bloodstream to combat infection.
- Releases a substance called "bile" to help digest food and absorb important nutrients.

Chapter 2: What is Fatty Liver Disease?

Fatty Liver disease develops over time and we are normally indirectly or directly the culprit for its development.

It is the build- up of extra fat in the liver cells. If more than 5% to 10% of the liver's weight is fatty, then it is called fatty liver—steatosis. On the other hand, should your liver become inflamed, this is called steatohepatitis. Once there is a build-up of fat the liver does becoming vulnerable to inflammation and scarring.

Fatty liver disease tends to develop in people who are overweight or obese or have diabetes, high cholesterol or high triglycerides/ lipids. This is a result of defective fatty acid metabolism and is normally caused by poor eating habits, too much alcohol or even certain medications. Therefore, fatty liver disease is divided into:

- Alcohol-related fatty liver disease (**ALD**).

- Non-alcoholic fatty liver disease (**NAFLD**).

That said, at least in the early stages, fatty liver disease doesn't present any overt symptoms, so you may not even realize you have it. For this reason, it's good to pay attention to what you eat and how much you drink and see your physician regularly.

Fatty Liver Disease is Reversible!

Remember the liver is very important. Without it we would poison ourselves. Although, there are currently no conventional medical treatments for Fatty Liver Disease, doctors may prescribe medicine that treat the contributing conditions such as insulin resistance, diabetes, high cholesterol or high triglycerides. Most cases, however, will simply call for lifestyle modification to implement a proper diet and regular cardiovascular exercise. Where alcohol is the principle cause, alcohol use should be discontinued immediately.

Chapter 3: Fatty Liver Disease Symptoms

Liver damage develops over time and most of the times we are directly or indirectly responsible for developing liver diseases.

When an inflammation occurs in the liver, it is called Hepatitis. When inflammation of the liver lasts longer than six months, the condition is called Chronic Hepatitis. Any sudden inflammation of the liver is called Acute Hepatitis.

If scar tissue is formed in the inflamed liver this is called Fibrosis. Fibrosis is something that is not sudden usually taking some time to develop. Think of it as over response. On the other hand when fibrosis and inflammation spread throughout the liver causing extensive scarring and disrupts its shape and function, this is called Cirrhosis .

Left unchecked cirrhosis can lead to liver cancer, liver failure or death. In other words, the body is essentially poisoned as all the chemicals and waste that liver was supposed to flush out, builds up in the body leading to organ failure and death in the worst case scenario.

In the nascent stages of fatty liver disease, symptoms can be asymptomatic or may include some of the following:

- Weight loss
- Nausea
- Tiredness
- Weakness
- Concentration problems
- Loss of appetite
- Inflammation of the liver

If left to progress such as in the case of alcoholic fatty liver disease, your liver may could become extensive scarred (cirrhosis). More symptoms that may appear are:

- Jaundice (yellow spots on your skin and eyes)
- Fluid buildup
- Liver failure
- Internal bleeding

Chapter 4: Fatty Liver Disease Diagnosis and Treatment

Fatty liver disease is usually diagnosed by your doctor at your routine checkup. By checking your abdomen your doctor might notice that your liver is larger than it should be.

By running certain tests your doctor can ascertain just what is happening.

Three common tests that your doctor uses are:

- **Blood tests**. A high number of certain enzymes could mean you've got fatty liver. These are the: Alanine transaminase (**ALT**) test and the Aspartate transaminase (**AST**) test. Consistently high levels of **ALT** can be a sign of liver swelling or injury. On the other hand, high levels **of AST** can be a sign of liver damage.
- **Ultrasound**. It uses soundwaves to get a picture of your liver. The doctor may also call for a CT Scan / MRI for more reports. However, this is seldom done.
- **Biopsy.** After numbing the area, your doctor puts a needle through your skin and takes out a tiny piece of liver. He looks at it under a microscope for signs of fat, inflammation, and damaged liver cells.

Treatment of Fatty Liver Disease

Although there is no specific treatment, you can improve your condition by managing your diabetes, if you have it. That said, sometimes doctors prescribe medicine that treat the contributing conditions such as insulin resistance, diabetes, high cholesterol or high triglycerides.

If you have alcoholic liver disease and you are a heavy drinker, quitting is the most important thing you can do. Talk to your doctor about how to get help. If you don't stop you could get complications like alcoholic hepatitis or cirrhosis.

Even if you have nonalcoholic fatty liver disease, it can help to avoid drinking. Remember drinking is sugar. If you are overweight or obese, do what you can to gradually lose weight -- no more than 1 or 2 pounds a week.

Lastly, eat a balanced and healthy diet and get regular exercise. Limit high-carb foods such as bread, grits, rice, potatoes, and corn. And cut down on drinks with lots of sugar like sports drinks and juice.

Chapter 5: Fatty Liver Disease What to Avoid, Limit and Eliminate

In understanding fatty liver disease, it is important to recognize just exactly what contributes to its development. What can I eat? What can't I eat? Do I have to starve myself and be a skeleton at the feast?

Let's drill down a bit and quickly cover the groups that have been linked to Fatty Liver Disease:

- **Cholesterol Foods** - High cholesterol is a factor that may elevate your risk of developing liver disease. Cholesterol, a type of fat, is only found in animal products. It is highest in fatty red meats, shrimp, egg yolks, cream, butter and organ meats.

- **Fatty Foods** - High-fat foods contribute to high cholesterol, high triglycerides and obesity when consumed in excess amounts, which the American Liver Foundation states are liver disease risk factors. Examples of high-fat foods include lard, shortening, butter, margarine, fat from meat, cream, cheese, chicken skin, deep-fried foods, creamy salad dressings, baked goods, desserts, pastries and mayonnaise.

- **Alcoholic Beverages** - Consuming excessive amounts of alcohol can lead to liver malfunction. If you drink alcohol then you should do so in moderation, which is defined as 2 drinks a day for men. If you already have liver disease or a malfunctioning liver, you should avoid all alcoholic beverages to prevent disease progression.

- **Sugary Foods** - Sugary products such as soda, candy and desserts tend to be high in calories. The United States Department of Agriculture notes that excess calorie consumption is a risk factor for liver disease and a major cause of obesity. Sugary foods should be portioned to prevent overeating and only consumed on occasion.

Chapter 6: Lifestyle and Diet Changes

The most effective way to treat the causes of and fatty liver disease is by making certain diet and lifestyle changes such as:

- Limiting alcoholic beverages and drinks sweetened with fruit sugar (fructose). Instead, drink plenty of nonalcoholic beverages, especially water.

- Exercising regularly and losing weight. Keeping your body at a healthy weight reduces your risk of a fatty liver condition.

- Limiting Sugary products such as candy and desserts that tend to be high in calories. The United States Department of Agriculture notes that excess calorie consumption is a risk factor for liver disease and a major cause of obesity.

High-Fructose Corn Syrup (HFCS)

Although fatty liver disease is commonly blamed on eating too many deserts and what we have deemed junk food, there is another clear culprit— high-fructose corn syrup.

Countless health problems have been linked to the consumption of high fructose corn syrup, not the least of which is fatty liver disease. A recent study showed that consumption of sugar-sweetened soft drinks is strongly associated with an increased risk of developing diabetes and fatty liver.

The study, done by U.S. and Canadian researchers, indicated that men who drank two or more sugary soft drinks a day had an 83 percent higher risk of fatty liver than those who drank less than one a month. In fact, the risk significantly increased among men who drank five to six servings of sugary soft drinks a week.

This makes sense on many levels, but first and foremost because Fructose reduces the affinity of insulin for its receptor, which is the principle characteristic of type 2 diabetes. Furthermore, High Fructose Corn Syrup has been implicated in elevated blood cholesterol levels, and it has been found to inhibit the action of white blood cells in your immune system.

Many of the health conditions that HFCS causes including high cholesterol, diabetes, also increase your risk of developing fatty liver disease. Additionally, fructose converts more readily to fat than other sugars, making it a major risk factor for both diabetes and obesity.

In a fructose metabolism study, it was noted that when two high-fructose breakfast drinks were consumed, the build-up of stored fat continued into the afternoon, during which time the quick conversion of fructose to fat remained active during digestion of the lunch meal. The study concluded that the higher the concentration of fructose in the diet, the higher the rate of fat conversion.

Frequently, fruit juices also have fructose added to them, and if you still believe that this is an acceptable form of sugar, think again. Fructose contains no beneficial enzymes, vitamins, minerals, or additional micronutrients. Instead, it actually leeches them from your body. Unbound fructose, found in large quantities in high fructose corn syrup, can also interfere with your heart's use of vital minerals such as magnesium, copper, and chromium.

Look At the Labels

You may think that avoiding fructose means just staying stay away from desserts and sweet drinks, but unfortunately there is more to it as fructose is hidden in many foods you would not even suspect. Names such as:: 'chicory,' 'inulin,' 'iso glucose,' 'glucose-fructose syrup,' 'dahlia syrup,' 'tapioca syrup,' 'glucose syrup,' 'corn syrup,' 'crystalline fructose,' and flat-out fraud 'fruit fructose,' or... 'agave'. Even processed meats and other foods you would never imagine contain high fructose corn syrup.

Limiting or Eliminating Alcohol is Crucial to Successful Fatty Liver Treatment

Fatty Liver is often seen in association with hypertension, excessive alcohol consumption, and coronary artery disease, so alcohol is a strong risk factor for this disease. In general, I believe alcohol should be reserved for people who have already achieved optimal wellness and therefore have their carbohydrates (sugars and grains) under control, and do not have disease conditions such as fatty liver, diabetes, or other signs of ill health.

Although wine has been shown to have some health benefits, it may also increase your insulin levels, which is not only a risk factor for diabetes, but increased insulin levels have been linked with a shorter life span, in general. So it needs to be used cautiously.

Drink Water

Drink plenty of water to help flush the system. To counter dehydration & hunger, drink 8, 8 oz glasses of water per day.

Exercise Can Dramatically Help

Exercise is needed as a necessary adjunct to a healthier lifestyle. Exercise will even help to prevent fatty liver by increasing circulation and normalizing your blood sugar levels, which it does primarily by normalizing your insulin levels.

An exercise routine has other advantages as well. Studies have shown that it works as an effective antidepressant, strengthens your immune system so it can fight off diseases like cancer, and it can even improve insulin resistance and reverse pre-diabetic conditions.

Maintaining Ideal Body Weight is a Large Part of the Solution

It seems to me, one of the greatest risk factors for fatty liver is obesity, or any excessive weight gain. Medical data shows a remarkably high prevalence of metabolic syndrome (heart disease and diabetes symptoms such as insulin resistance, abdominal obesity, hypertension, and high triglyceride levels) in people with fatty liver disease.

Weight loss represents a safe method for reducing inflammatory states. Remember fatty liver is an inflammatory condition, and it is clear that losing weight, and keeping it off, will greatly improve your chances or keeping your liver healthy.

Chapter 7: Breakfast

<u>Old Fashioned Scrambled Eggs</u>

Ingredients

- 8 eggs
- 1(5 ounce) can evaporated milk
- 2 tablespoons butter
- salt and pepper for taste

Directions

1. In a bowl, whisk the eggs and milk until combined.
2. In a skillet, heat butter until hot.
3. Add egg mixture; cook and stir over medium-low heat until eggs are completely set.
4. Season with salt and pepper.

<u>Baked Apple Oatmeal</u>

Ingredients

- 2 2/3 cups old-fashioned oats
- ½ cup raisins
- 4 cups milk
- 2 tablespoons butter or margarine, melted
- 1 teaspoon ground cinnamon
- ¼ teaspoon salt
- 2 medium apples, chopped (2 cups)

Directions

1. 1 Heat oven to 350°F. In 2-quart casserole, mix oats, raisins, 4 cups milk, the brown sugar, butter, cinnamon, salt and apples.

2. 2 Bake uncovered 40 to 45 minutes or until most liquid is absorbed. Top with walnuts. Serve with additional milk.

Zucchini & Eggs

Ingredients

- 4 eggs, lightly beaten
- 2 tablespoons grated Parmesan cheese
- 2 tablespoons olive oil
- 1 zucchini, sliced 1/8- to 1/4-inch thick
- garlic powder or salt
- ground black pepper to taste

Directions

1. Stir the eggs and Parmesan cheese together in a bowl; set aside.
2. Heat the olive oil in a large skillet over medium-high heat; cook the zucchini in the hot oil until softened and lightly browned, about 7 minutes. Season the zucchini with garlic powder, salt, and pepper. Reduce heat to medium; pour the egg mixture into the skillet. Cook, stirring gently, for about 3 minutes.
3. Remove the skillet from the heat and cover. Keep covered off the heat until the eggs set, about 2 minutes more and serve.

Morning Green Smoothie

Ingredients

- 1 cucumber, sliced
- 2 kiwi fruits, peeled and sliced

- 1 cup baby spinach
- 1 cup coconut milk
- 2 tablespoons raw honey
- 1 pinch ground ginger

Directions

1. Combine all the ingredients in a blender and pulse until smooth and creamy.
2. Pour the mixture into glasses and serve right away.

Cinnamon Carrot Baked Oatmeal

Ingredients

- 2 cups rolled oats
- ¼ teaspoon cinnamon powder
- ¼ teaspoon ground ginger
- ½ cup walnuts, chopped
- 2 carrots, grated
- ¼ cup maple syrup
- ¼ cup dates, pitted and chopped
- 2 cups coconut milk
- 2 tablespoons raw honey

Directions

1. Combine all the ingredients in a deep dish baking pan.
2. Cook in the preheated oven at 350F for 10-15 minutes until softened.
3. Serve the oatmeal warm.

Mom's Eggs Benedict

Ingredients

- 4 slices Canadian bacon
- 1 teaspoon white vinegar
- 4 eggs
- 1 cup butter
- 3 egg yolks
- 1 tablespoon heavy cream
- 1 dash ground cayenne pepper
- ½ teaspoon salt
- 1 tablespoon lemon juice
- 4 whole wheat English muffins, split and toasted

Directions

1. In a skillet over medium-high heat, fry the Canadian bacon on each side until evenly browned.
2. Fill a large saucepan with about 3 inches water, and bring to a simmer. Pour in the vinegar. Carefully break the 4 eggs into the water, and cook 2 to 3 minutes, until whites are set but yolks are still soft. Remove eggs with a slotted spoon.
3. Meanwhile, melt the butter until bubbly in a small pan or in the microwave. Remove from heat before butter browns.
4. In a blender or large food processor, blend the egg yolks, heavy cream, cayenne pepper, and salt until smooth. Add half of the hot butter in a thin steady stream, slow enough so that it blends in at least as fast as you are pouring it in. Blend in the lemon juice using the same method, then the remaining butter.
5. Place open English muffins onto serving plates. Top with 1 slice Canadian bacon and 1 poached egg. Drizzle with the cream sauce, and serve at once.

Pumpkin Pancakes

Ingredients

- 1 ¼ cups all-purpose flour
- 2 tablespoons sugar
- 2 teaspoons baking powder
- ½ teaspoon cinnamon
- ½ teaspoon ginger
- ½ teaspoon nutmeg
- ½ teaspoon salt
- 1 pinch clove
- 1 cup 1% low-fat milk
- 6 tablespoons canned pumpkin puree
- 2 tablespoons melted butter
- 1 egg

Directions

1. Whisk flour, sugar, baking powder, spices and salt in a bowl.
2. In a separate bowl whisk together milk, pumpkin, melted butter, and egg.
3. Fold mixture into dry ingredients.
4. Spray or grease a skillet and heat over medium heat: pour in 1/ 4 cup batter for each pancake.
5. Cook pancakes about 3 minutes per side. Serve with butter and syrup. Makes about six 6-inch pancakes.

Cornflakes with Berries

Ingredients

1. 2 cups cornflakes
2. 1 cup 1% low-fat milk
3. 1 cup berries, fresh or frozen, thawed

Directions

1. Place cornflakes in a small bowl.
2. Top with milk and berries and serve.

Berry Breakfast Quinoa

Ingredients:

- ¼ cup milk
- 2 containers (6 oz each) 99% Fat Free French vanilla, strawberry or peach yogurt
- 4 teaspoons chia seed
- 1 cup cooled cooked quinoa (1/4 cup uncooked)
- 2 cups fresh fruit (mixed berries or chopped peaches)
- ¼ cup coarsely chopped toasted almonds or pecans
- 1/8 teaspoon ground cinnamon

Directions:

1. In medium bowl, stir together milk, yogurt and chia seed until blended. Evenly divide mixture among 4 glasses. Spoon 1/4 cup cooled cooked quinoa on top of yogurt layer on each.
2. Top each with a layer of fruit and almonds. Sprinkle with cinnamon. Let stand 5 minutes, or cover and refrigerate overnight.

Banana-Blueberry Smoothie

Ingredients:

- 1 cup milk
- 1 cup Cheerios cereal
- 1 ripe banana, cut into chunks

- 1 cup fresh blueberries
- 1 cup ice
- Garnishes, If Desired
- Banana slices
- Additional cereal

Directions:

1. In blender, place Smoothie ingredients. Cover; blend on high speed about 30 seconds or until smooth.
2. Pour into 2 glasses. Garnish as desired. Serve immediately.

Cherry Strawberry Smoothie

Ingredients:

- 2 containers (5.3 oz each) honey Greek yogurt
- 1 ½ cups frozen organic cherries
- ½ cup frozen organic strawberries
- 1 cup milk

Directions:

1. In blender, place all ingredients. Cover and blend on high speed about 1 minute or until smooth.
2. Pour into 3 glasses. Serve immediately.

Orange Flaxseed Smoothie

Ingredients

- 2 oranges, cut into segments
- 2 peaches, pitted and sliced
- 1 cup carrot juice

- ¼ teaspoon cinnamon powder
- 1 pinch ground ginger
- 2 tablespoons ground flaxseeds

Directions

1. Combine all the ingredients in a blender. Pulse until smooth and creamy.
2. Serve the smoothie fresh and chilled.

Chapter 8: Salads

Winter Fruit Waldorf Salad

Ingredients:

- 2 medium unpeeled red apples, diced
- 2 medium unpeeled pears, diced
- ½ cup thinly sliced celery
- ½ cup golden raisins
- ½ cup chopped dates
- ¼ cup gluten-free mayonnaise or salad dressing
- ¼ cup 99% Fat Free orange crème yogurt (from 6-oz container)
- 2 tablespoons frozen orange juice concentrate
- 8 cups shredded lettuce
- Walnut halves, if desired

Directions:

1. In large bowl, mix apples, pears, celery, raisins and dates.
2. In small bowl, mix mayonnaise, yogurt and juice concentrate until well blended. Add to fruit; toss to coat. (Salad can be refrigerated up to 1 hour.) Serve on lettuce. Garnish with walnut halves.

Quinoa and Vegetable Salad

Ingredients:

- 1 cup uncooked quinoa
- 2 tablespoons fresh lemon juice
- 2 tablespoons olive oil
- 2 tablespoons chopped fresh basil
- 1 can (15 oz) gluten-free garbanzo beans, drained, rinsed

- 1 can (15.25 oz) gluten-free whole kernel sweet corn, drained
- 1 can (14.5 oz) gluten-free diced tomatoes, drained
- 1 cup chopped red bell pepper
- 1/3 cup quartered pitted olives
- ½ cup crumbled gluten-free feta cheese

Directions:

1. Rinse quinoa under cold water 1 minute; drain. Cook quinoa as directed on package; drain. Cool completely, about 30 minutes.
2. Meanwhile, in small nonmetal bowl, place lemon juice, oil and basil; mix well. Set aside for dressing.
3. In large bowl, gently toss cooked quinoa, beans, corn, tomatoes, bell pepper and olives. Pour dressing over quinoa mixture; toss gently to coat. Serve immediately or refrigerate 1 to 2 hours before serving.

Garden Citrus Salad

Ingredients

- 2 cups baby spinach
- 2 cups arugula leaves
- 1 zucchini, sliced
- 1 red onion, sliced
- 2 tablespoons chopped cilantro
- 1 orange, cut into segments
- 1 lime, juiced
- 2 tablespoons extra virgin olive oil
- Salt and pepper

Directions

1. Combine the baby spinach, arugula leaves, zucchini, red onion, cilantro and orange in a salad bowl.
2. Drizzle in the lime juice and oil then season with salt and pepper. Serve the salad fresh.

Zesty Garden Salad

Ingredients

- 1 teaspoon Dijon mustard
- 1 sprig fresh dill, chopped (optional)
- 1 tablespoon chopped green onion
- 2 tablespoons shredded Cheddar cheese
- ½ cup sweet corn kernels
- ½ cup sugar snap peas
- 1/3 cup frozen shelled edamame (optional)
- 2 cups iceberg lettuce
- 1 pinch salt and pepper

Directions

1. Stir the Dijon mustard, dill, green onion, Cheddar cheese, corn, peas, and edamame in a bowl until evenly combined.
2. Stir in the iceberg lettuce, season to taste with salt and pepper, and toss to mix.

Orange & Duck Confit Salad

Ingredients

- 1 tablespoon sherry vinegar

- 4 blood oranges, divided (3 sectioned, about 1 cup; 1 juiced, about 1/ 4 cup)
- 1 teaspoon Dijon mustard
- 1 tablespoon olive oil
- ¼ teaspoon salt
- ¼ teaspoon pepper
- 1 small duck confit leg (5-6 ounces), shredded, skin, fat, and bones discarded (about 3/ 4 cup)
- 6 cups mixed winter salad greens (such as romaine, escarole, and spinach)
- ¼ cup skinned chopped hazelnuts, toasted

Directions

1. In a small bowl, combine vinegar, orange juice, mustard, and oil, whisking well. Whisk in salt and pepper.
2. In a large bowl, combine shredded duck, salad greens, hazelnuts, and orange sections. Drizzle with vinaigrette; serve.

Mom's Potato Salad

Ingredients

- 2 potatoes
- 1 sweet potato
- 4 eggs
- 2 stalks celery, chopped
- ½ onion, chopped
- ¾ cup mayonnaise
- 1 tablespoon prepared mustard
- 1 teaspoon salt
- 1 ½ teaspoons ground black pepper

Directions

1. Bring a large pot of salted water to a boil. Add potatoes and cook until tender but still firm, about 30 minutes. Drain, cool, peel and chop.
2. Place eggs in a saucepan and cover with cold water. Bring water to a boil. Cover, remove from heat, and let eggs stand in hot water for 10 to 12 minutes. Remove from hot water; cool, peel and chop.
3. Combine the potatoes, eggs, celery and onion. Whisk together the mayonnaise, mustard, salt and pepper. Add to potato mixture, toss well to coat. Refrigerate and serve chilled.

Strawberry-Spinach Salad

Ingredients

- 3 cups baby spinach
- 1 cup strawberries, halved
- 1 red onion, sliced
- 1 can of tuna
- 1 tablespoon white wine vinegar
- 1 tablespoon lemon juice
- 1 teaspoon mustard
- 2 tablespoons extra virgin olive oil

Directions

1. Combine the spinach, strawberries, red onion and tuna in a salad bowl.
2. For the dressing, mix the vinegar, lemon juice, mustard and olive oil in a bowl. Add salt and pepper to taste and mix well.
3. Drizzle the dressing over the salad and serve it fresh.

Cherry Tomato Corn Salad

Ingredients

- ¼ cup minced fresh basil
- 3 tablespoons olive oil
- 2 teaspoons lime juice
- 1 teaspoon sugar
- ½ teaspoon salt
- ¼ teaspoon pepper
- 2 cups frozen corn, thawed
- 2 cups cherry tomatoes, halved
- 1 cup chopped seeded and peeled cucumber

Directions

1. In a jar with a tight-fitting lid, combine the basil, oil, lime juice, sugar, salt and pepper; shake well.
2. In a large bowl, combine the corn, tomatoes and cucumber.
3. Drizzle with dressing and toss to coat. Refrigerate until serving.

Summer Watermelon Salad

Ingredients

- ¼ cup balsamic vinegar
- 1 tablespoon Dijon mustard
- 1 tablespoon chopped garlic
- ½ teaspoon salt
- ½ teaspoon freshly ground black pepper
- ¾ cup olive oil
- 3 cups 2-inch cubes watermelon
- 1 cup crumbled feta cheese
- ½ red onion, sliced very thin

- coarsely ground black pepper for taste

Directions

1. Mix the vinegar and Dijon mustard in a bowl. Stir the garlic, salt, and pepper into the mixture. Slowly stream the olive oil into the dressing while whisking vigorously. Place the dressing in the refrigerator until ready to use.
2. Combine the watermelon, feta cheese, and red onion in a large bowl; toss lightly to mix. Season with the coarsely ground black pepper.
3. Pour about half the dressing over the salad; gently toss to coat. Refrigerate the salad at least 30 minutes. Drizzle the remaining dressing over the salad just before serving.

<u>Spinach Grapefruit Salad</u>

Ingredients

- 4 cups baby spinach
- 2 grapefruits, cut into segments
- 1 red onion, sliced
- ¼ cup hazelnuts, chopped
- ½ cup plain yogurt
- 2 tablespoons lemon juice
- 2 tablespoons extra virgin olive oil
- Salt and pepper for taste

Directions

1. Combine the baby spinach, grapefruits, onion and hazelnuts in a bowl.
2. Combine the yogurt, lemon juice, olive oil, salt and pepper in a glass jar.
3. Shake until creamy.
4. Drizzle the dressing over the salad and serve it fresh.

Chunky Vegetable Salad

Ingredients

- 4 tomatoes, cubes
- 1 cup cooked chickpeas, drained
- 1 jalapeno pepper, chopped
- 1 red bell pepper, cored and diced
- 1 celery stalk, sliced
- 1 cucumber, sliced
- 2 tablespoons olive oil
- 1 tablespoon balsamic vinegar
- 1 tablespoon chopped parsley
- 1 tablespoon chopped cilantro
- Add a pinch of salt and pepper.

Directions

1. Combine all the ingredients in a salad bowl.
2. Add salt and pepper and serve the salad warm and fresh.

Chapter 9: Soups & Appetizers

Roasted Garlic & Cauliflower Soup

Ingredients

- 1 large head cauliflower (about 2 ½ lb.)
- 4 ½ teaspoons olive oil
- 1 ½ teaspoons kosher salt
- 3 garlic cloves, divided & unpeeled
- 3 cups chicken broth
- 1 cup 2% reduced-fat milk
- ½ cup grated Parmesan cheese
- Freshly ground black pepper
- Garnishes: olive oil, pomegranate seeds, fresh thyme leaves

Directions

1. Preheat oven to 425 °. Cut cauliflower into 2-inch florets; toss with olive oil and 1/ 2 tsp. salt. Arrange florets in a single layer on a jelly-roll pan. Wrap garlic cloves in aluminum foil, and place on jelly-roll pan with cauliflower.
2. Bake at 425 ° for 30 to 40 minutes or until cauliflower is golden brown, tossing cauliflower every 15 minutes.
3. Transfer cauliflower to a large Dutch oven. Unwrap garlic, and cool 5 minutes. Peel garlic, and add to cauliflower. Add stock, and bring to a simmer over medium heat; simmer, stirring occasionally, 5 minutes. Let mixture cool 10 minutes.
4. Process cauliflower mixture, in batches, in a blender until smooth, stopping to scrape down sides as needed.
5. Return cauliflower mixture to Dutch oven; stir in milk, cheese, and remaining 1 tsp. salt. Cook over low heat,

stirring occasionally, 2 to 3 minutes or until thoroughly heated. Add pepper for taste.

Lentil Soup

Ingredients:

- 1 cup regular lentils
- ¼ cup wild rice
- ¼ cup barley,
- 4 cups vegetable broth
- 2 cups chopped kale
- sea salt, pepper

Directions:

1. In a large pot, add the broth and let it boil.
2. Add the rest of the ingredients and seasoning.
3. Cover and let it simmer for about 40 min.
4. Add the kale and let it cook for about 15 more min.

Carrot Soup

Ingredients:

- 2 bags (1 lb each) ready-to-eat baby-cut carrots
- 2 large onions, chopped (about 2 cups)
- 5 ¼ cups chicken broth (from two 32-oz cartons)
- ½ teaspoon salt
- ½ cup whipping cream
- ½ cup orange juice
- 3 tablespoons packed brown sugar
- 2 tablespoons grated gingerroot
- ¼ teaspoon white pepper
- Fresh orange slices, quartered, if desired

- Fresh Italian parsley, if desired

Directions:

1. Spray 4- to 5-quart slow cooker with cooking spray. In cooker, mix carrots, onions, broth and salt.
2. Cover; cook on Low heat setting 8 to 10 hours.
3. Pour 4 cups of the soup mixture to blender; add half each of the whipping cream, orange juice, brown sugar, gingerroot and pepper. Cover and blend until smooth; return to cooker. Blend remaining soup mixture with remaining half of ingredients; return to cooker.
4. Increase heat setting to High. Cover; cook 15 to 20 minutes longer or until hot. Garnish individual servings with an orange quarter and parsley.

Home-Style Potato Soup

Ingredients

- 3 medium potatoes (about 1 pound)
- 1 ¾ cups chicken broth (from 32-ounce carton)
- 2 medium green onions with tops
- 1 ½ cups milk
- ¼ teaspoon salt
- 1/8 teaspoon pepper
- 1/8 teaspoon dried thyme leaves

Directions

1. Peel the potatoes, and cut into large pieces.
2. Heat the chicken broth and potatoes to boiling in the saucepan over high heat, stirring occasionally with a fork to make sure potatoes do not stick to the saucepan. Once mixture is boiling, reduce heat just enough so mixture bubbles gently. Cover and cook about 15 minutes or until potatoes are tender when pierced with a fork.

3. While the potatoes are cooking, peel and thinly slice the green onions. If you have extra onions, wrap them airtight and store in the refrigerator up to 5 days.
4. When the potatoes are done, remove the saucepan from the heat, but do not drain. Break the potatoes into smaller pieces with the potato masher or large fork. The mixture should still be lumpy.
5. Stir the milk, salt, pepper, thyme and onions into the potato mixture. Heat over medium heat, stirring occasionally, until hot and steaming, but do not let the soup boil.

Greek Cold Cucumber Soup

Ingredients

- 4 cucumbers
- 2 cups plain yogurt
- 2 garlic cloves
- Salt and pepper
- 2 tablespoons lemon juice
- 2 tablespoons chopped dill

Directions

1. Combine the cucumbers, yogurt, garlic, lemon juice, salt and pepper in a blender.
2. Pulse until smooth.
3. Stir in the dill and serve the soup chilled.

Gazpacho

Ingredients

- 1 hothouse cucumber. halved and seeded, but not peeled
- 2 red bell peppers, cored and seeded
- 4 plum tomatoes

- 1 red onion
- 2 garlic cloves, minced
- 3 cups tomato juice
- ¼ cup white wine vinegar
- ¼ cup olive oil
- ½ tablespoon salt
- 1 teaspoon freshly ground black pepper

Directions

1. Roughly chop the cucumbers, bell peppers, tomatoes, and red onions into 1-inch cubes.
2. Put each vegetable separately into a food processor fitted with a steel blade and pulse until it is coarsely chopped.
3. Once each vegetable is processed, combine them in a large bowl and add the garlic, tomato juice, vinegar, olive oil, salt, and pepper. Mix well and chill before serving.

Mint Ginger Sweet Potato Soup

Ingredients

- 1 tablespoon olive oil
- 2 medium-large sweet potatos peeled, chopped, and pureed
- 1 clove garlic
- 1 teaspoon ginger
- 1/ 3 teaspoon turmeric
- 4 diced mint leaves
- 2 cups vegetable broth

Directions

1. Pour olive oil into food processor.
2. Add the washed, peeled and pieces of sweet potato into the food processor with the oil.

3. Add garlic clove to the food processor.
4. Add the ginger turmeric.
5. Wash, dry, and chop mint leaves.
6. Puree.
7. Pour into medium sized pot or Dutch oven.
8. Add broth.
9. Let sit over medium heat for 25-30 minutes.

Creamy Garlic Zucchini Soup

Ingredients

- 2 tablespoons extra virgin olive oil
- 4 garlic cloves, chopped
- 1 shallot, chopped
- 3 zucchinis, cubed
- 2 potatoes, peeled and cubed
- 2 cups water
- 2 cups vegetable stock
- Salt and pepper to taste

Directions:

1. Heat the oil in a soup pot and add the garlic and shallot.
2. Cook for a few seconds then add the rest of the ingredients.
3. Season with salt and pepper and cook on low heat for 15 minutes.
4. When done, puree the soup with an immersion blender.
5. Pour the soup into serving bowls

Vegetables & Hummus

Ingredients

- ¾ cup mixed vegetables, such as baby carrots, cherry tomatoes and red bell pepper slices
- 1 (15.5 ounce) can garbanzo beans (chickpeas), drained 1/3 cup pitted Spanish Manzanilla olives
- 1 teaspoon minced garlic
- 3 tablespoons olive oil
- 2 tablespoons lemon juice
- 1 ½ teaspoons chopped fresh basil
- 1 teaspoon cilantro leaves
- salt and pepper for taste

Directions

1. Wash vegetables and a slice them into bitable sizes.
2. Place garbanzo beans, olives, and garlic into the bowl of a blender or food processor. Pour in olive oil and lemon juice; season with basil, cilantro, salt, and pepper.
3. Cover and puree until smooth.
4. Arrange vegetables on a platter.
5. Dip into hummus and eat.

Deviled Eggs

Ingredients

- 12 eggs 1 jalapeno pepper, minced
- 1 habanero peppers, seeded and minced
- ¼ cup mayonnaise
- 1 teaspoon yellow mustard
- 1/8 teaspoon paprika

Directions

1. Place the eggs into a saucepan in a single layer, and fill with water to cover the eggs by at least 1 inch. Bring the water to a boil over high heat. Cover, and remove from the heat; let the eggs stand in the hot water for 15 minutes. Pour out the hot water, then cool the eggs under cold running water in the sink. Peel.

2. Cut the cooled eggs in half lengthwise. Remove the yolks, and place them into a mixing bowl along with the jalapeno, habanero, mayonnaise, and mustard; mash together until smooth. Transfer the yolk mixture to a pastry bag, and decoratively squeeze into the white halves. Sprinkle with paprika to garnish.

Zucchini Boats

Ingredients

- 2 zucchinis
- 1 pound ground chicken
- 1 teaspoon dried basil
- 1 teaspoon dried oregano
- 2 tablespoons chopped parsley
- 1 shallot, chopped
- Salt and pepper for taste
- 1 cup tomato sauce
- ½ cup dry white wine
- 1 bay leaf

Directions

1. Cut the zucchinis in half and carefully scoop out the flesh. Chop the zucchini flesh finely and place it in a bowl.

2. Add the ground chicken, basil, oregano, parsley and shallot and season with salt and pepper. Spoon the mixture back into the zucchini boats.
3. Place the zucchini in a deep dish baking tray and pour in the tomato sauce and wine.
4. Add the bay leaf and a pinch of salt and pepper.
5. Cook in the preheated oven at 350F for 15-20 minutes.
6. Serve the zucchini boats warm.

Caprese Appetizer

Ingredients

- 20 grape tomatoes
- 10 ounces mozzarella cheese, cubed
- 2 tablespoons extra virgin olive oil
- 2 tablespoons fresh basil leaves, chopped
- 1 pinch salt
- 1 pinch ground black pepper
- 20 toothpicks

Directions

1. Toss tomatoes, mozzarella cheese, olive oil, basil, salt, and pepper together in a bowl until well coated.
2. Skewer one tomato and one piece of mozzarella cheese on each toothpick.

Kale & Tofu

Ingredients

- 3 oz. fresh kale leaves
- 3 oz. firm tofu cubes
- Olive oil for drizzling
- No-salt seasoning

Directions

1. Prepare baking tray and preheat oven to 400.
2. Layout individual kale leaves, drop one tofu cube in the center. Fold leaf ends over tofu cube and flip.
3. Drizzle with olive oil and seasoning Bake 18-22 minutes.

Minestrone Soup

Ingredients

- 2 tablespoons extra virgin olive oil
- 1 shallot, chopped 1 red bell pepper, cored and diced
- 2 carrots, diced
- 1 parsnip, diced
- 1 celery stalk, sliced
- 1 zucchini, cubed
- 2 cups green beans, chopped
- ½ cup green peas
- 2 cups baby spinach
- 1 cup diced tomatoes
- 4 cups water
- 2 cups vegetable stock
- ½ teaspoon dried oregano
- ½ teaspoon dried basil
- Salt and pepper to taste

Directions

1. Combine the olive oil and the vegetables in a soup pot.
2. Add the water, stock and herbs, as well as salt and pepper and cook on medium heat for 20-25 minutes.
3. Serve the soup warm and fresh, although it taste just as good chilled.

Chapter 10: Chicken

Asparagus Chicken Divan

Ingredients

- 1 pound skinless, boneless
- chicken breast halves
- 2 pounds fresh asparagus, trimmed
- 1 (10.75 ounce) can condensed cream of chicken soup, undiluted
- 1 teaspoon Worcestershire sauce
- ¼ teaspoon ground nutmeg
- 1 cup grated Parmesan cheese,
- ½ cup whipping cream, whipped
- ¾ cup mayonnaise*

Directions

1. Broil chicken 6 in. from the heat until juices run clear.
2. Meanwhile, in a large skillet, bring 1/2 in. of water to a boil. Add asparagus. Reduce heat; cover and simmer for 3-5 minutes or until crisp and tender.
3. Drain and place in a greased shallow 2-1/2-qt. baking dish.
4. Cut chicken into thin slices. In a bowl, combine the soup, Worcestershire sauce and nutmeg. Spread half over asparagus. Sprinkle with 1/3 cup Parmesan cheese. Top with chicken. Spread remaining soup mixture over chicken; sprinkle with 1/3 cup Parmesan cheese.
5. Bake, uncovered, at 400 degrees F for 20 minutes. Fold whipped cream into mayonnaise; spread over top. Sprinkle with remaining Parmesan cheese. Broil 4-6 in. from the heat for about 2 minutes or until golden brown.

Balsamic Chicken Breasts

Ingredients

- 2 sweet potatoes, peeled and cut into 2-inch pieces
- 1 tablespoon olive oil
- 2 skinless, boneless chicken breast halves
- ½ cup balsamic vinegar salt and ground black pepper for taste
- ½ cup balsamic vinegar

Directions

1. Preheat oven to 400 degrees F (200 degrees C).
2. Place the potatoes on a baking sheet; drizzle olive oil over potatoes and season with salt and pepper.
3. Place the chicken breasts in a baking dish. Pour 1/2 cup of balsamic vinegar over the breasts; season with salt and pepper. Cover with aluminum foil. Place the potatoes in the preheated oven and bake for 10 minutes; place the dish with the chicken in the oven and cook both the potatoes and chicken another 20 minutes; flip both the potatoes and chicken; reduce the oven heat to 350 degrees F (175 degrees C).
4. Bake another 20 minutes.
5. Pour ½ cup of balsamic vinegar into a small saucepan and place over medium heat. Cook until reduced to about ¼ cup. Place the chicken breasts atop the potatoes; drizzle with the reduced balsamic vinegar to serve.

Caribbean-Spiced Roast Chicken

Ingredients

- 1 ½ tablespoons fresh lime juice
- 2 fluid ounces rum
- 1 tablespoon brown sugar
- ¼ teaspoon cayenne pepper
- ¼ teaspoon ground clove
- ½ teaspoon ground cinnamon
- ½ teaspoon ground ginger
- 1 teaspoon black pepper
- ½ teaspoon salt
- ½ teaspoon dried thyme leaves
- 1 (3 pound) whole chicken
- 1 tablespoon vegetable oil

Directions

1. Preheat oven to 325 degrees F (165 degrees C).
2. In a small bowl, combine the lime juice, rum, and brown sugar; set aside. Mix together the cayenne pepper, clove, cinnamon, ginger, pepper, salt, and thyme leaves. Brush the chicken with oil, then coat with the spice mixture.
3. Place in a roasting pan, and bake about 90 minutes, until the juices run clear or until a meat thermometer inserted in thickest part of the thigh reaches 180 degrees F. Baste the chicken with the sauce every 20 minutes while it's cooking. Allow chicken to rest for 10 minutes before carving.

Sage and Garlic Grilled Chicken Breasts

Ingredients:

- 1 teaspoon dried sage leaves

- ½ teaspoon seasoned salt
- ½ teaspoon dried marjoram leaves
- ¼ teaspoon coarse ground black pepper
- 2 garlic cloves, minced
- 2 tablespoons olive oil
- 4 boneless skinless chicken breast halves

Directions:

1. Heat closed contact grill for 5 minutes.
2. Meanwhile, in small bowl, combine all ingredients except chicken breast halves; mix well. Place chicken on sheet of waxed paper. Brush or rub mixture onto all sides of chicken.
3. When grill is heated, place chicken on bottom grill surface. Close grill; cook 5 to 7 minutes or until chicken is fork-tender and juices run clear.

Herb & Garlic Chicken with Vegetables

Ingredients:

- 1 cut-up whole chicken (3 to 3 1/2 lb)
- 2 tablespoons olive or vegetable oil
- 1 envelope savory herb with garlic soup mix (from 2.4-oz box)
- 1/3 cup chicken broth
- 4 medium stalks celery, cut in half lengthwise, then cut into 4-inch pieces
- 1 large onion, cut into 6 wedges
- 2 large carrots, cut in half lengthwise, then cut into 4-inch pieces
- 2 medium unpeeled russet potatoes, each cut into 8 pieces

Directions:

1. Heat oven to 425°F. Remove skin from chicken if desired. In small bowl, mix oil, soup mix and broth. Brush both sides of chicken pieces with about half of the oil mixture.
2. In large bowl, mix celery, onion, carrots, potatoes and remaining oil mixture. Arrange vegetables in ungreased 15x10x1-inch pan. Bake 15 minutes.
3. Place chicken pieces in pan, overlapping vegetables if necessary. Bake 35 to 40 minutes longer or until vegetables are tender and juice of chicken is clear when thickest piece is cut to bone (170°F for breasts; 180°F for thighs and legs).

<u>Chicken Cacciatore</u>

Ingredients

- 6 chicken thighs
- 2 tablespoons extra virgin olive
- oil 1 sweet onion, chopped 2 garlic cloves, minced
- 2 red bell peppers, cored and diced
- 2 carrots, diced
- 1 rosemary sprig
- 1 thyme sprig
- 4 tomatoes, peeled and diced
- ½ cup tomato juice
- ¼ cup dry white wine
- 1 cup chicken stock
- Salt and pepper to taste
- 1 bay leaf

Directions

1. Heat the oil in a heavy saucepan.

2. Add the chicken and cook on all sides until golden.
3. Stir in the onion and garlic and cook for 2 minutes.
4. Stir in the rest of the ingredients and season with salt and pepper.
5. Cook on low heat for 30 minutes.
6. Serve the chicken cacciatore warm.

Chicken Marsala

Ingredients

- 4 chicken fillets
- 1 tablespoon cornstarch
- 2 tablespoons extra virgin olive oil
- 2 prosciutto slices, chopped
- 1 pound button mushrooms
- ¼ cup Marsala wine
- 1 cup chicken stock
- Salt and pepper to taste

Directions

1. Season the chicken with salt and pepper then sprinkle with cornstarch.
2. Heat the oil in a saucepan and place the chicken in the hot oil.
3. Cook on each side until golden then add the rest of the ingredients.
4. Season with salt and pepper and cook on low heat for 25 minutes.
5. Serve the chicken and the sauce warm.

Braised Chicken with Wild Mushrooms and Thyme

Ingredients

- 1 cup boiling water
- ½ oz dried porcini mushrooms
- 1 tablespoon butter
- 1 tablespoon olive oil
- 1 cut-up broiler-fryer chicken (3 to 3 1/2 lb)
- 2 large onions, chopped (2 cups)
- 5 cloves garlic, finely chopped
- 6 medium button mushrooms, sliced
- 2 medium carrots, chopped (1 cup)
- 2 medium stalks celery, chopped (1 cup)
- 2 dried bay leaves
- 2 fresh thyme sprigs or 1 teaspoon dried thyme leaves
- 5 tablespoons chopped fresh parsley
- 1 cup chicken broth
- ½ cup dry white wine or chicken broth
- 1 can (14.5 oz) diced tomatoes, undrained
- ¼ teaspoon salt
- ¼ teaspoon freshly ground pepper

Directions

1. Adjust oven rack to middle position. Heat oven to 300°F.
2. In small bowl, pour boiling water over dried mushrooms. Let stand 30 minutes to allow mushrooms to rehydrate (if mushrooms float to surface, place small saucer in bowl to keep them submerged). Use slotted spoon to remove rehydrated mushrooms from water; set aside. Reserve mushroom water.
3. In 4- or 5-quart ovenproof Dutch oven, heat butter and oil over medium-high heat until butter is melted. Add half of the chicken pieces and cook 6 minutes, turning occasionally, until chicken is deep golden brown (you are

not cooking the chicken, just giving it color). Remove chicken from Dutch oven and place on plate. Repeat with remaining chicken.

4.   Reduce heat to medium and add onions and garlic. Cook 5 minutes, stirring occasionally, until soft. Add rehydrated and sliced button mushrooms, carrots, celery, bay leaves, thyme and 3 tablespoons of the parsley. Cook 5 minutes, stirring occasionally, until vegetables are softened and mushrooms give up their juices.

5.   Add reserved mushroom water and heat to a simmer. Simmer uncovered 10 minutes (you are trying to concentrate the flavor of the liquid). Add chicken (along with any juices that may have accumulated on plate), broth, wine, tomatoes, salt and pepper.

6.   Cover pan and place in oven. Bake 1 1/2 hours or until chicken is very tender and there is a good amount of broth. Remove and discard bay leaves and thyme sprig. Place 2 pieces chicken into each of 4 large, flat serving bowls and ladle broth over. Sprinkle with remaining 2 tablespoons parsley.

Chapter 11: Turkey

Grilled Turkey Tenderloins

Ingredients

- ¼ cup reduced-sodium soy sauce
- 4 teaspoons canola oil
- 1 teaspoon sugar
- 1 garlic clove, minced
- ½ teaspoon ground ginger
- ½ teaspoon ground mustard
- ¾ pound turkey breast tenderloins

Directions

1. In a bowl, combine the soy sauce, oil, sugar, garlic, ginger and mustard. Pour 1/4 cup marinade into a large resealable plastic bag; add the turkey. Seal bag and turn to coat; refrigerate for up to 4 hours. Cover and refrigerate remaining marinade for basting.
2. Coat grill rack with nonstick cooking spray before starting the grill. Drain and discard marinade from turkey. Grill turkey, covered, over medium heat for 8-10 minutes or until a meat thermometer reads 170 degrees F, turning twice and basting occasionally with reserved marinade. Cut into slices.

Mom's Turkey Meatloaf

Ingredients

- 1 ½ pounds ground turkey
- 1 small onion, minced
- 2 stalks celery, minced
- 3 cloves garlic, minced
- 2 teaspoons chopped fresh basil

- ¼ cup Parmesan cheese
- ½ cup whole wheat bread crumbs
- 1 egg
- ¼ cup milk
- 1 (10.75 ounce) can condensed tomato soup

Directions

1. Preheat an oven to 350 degrees F (175 degrees C). Prepare a 9x13 inch baking dish with cooking spray.
2. Mix the ground turkey, onion, celery, garlic, basil, Parmesan cheese, bread crumbs, egg, and milk together in a large bowl. Shape the mixture into a loaf and place into prepared pan. Pour the tomato soup over the meatloaf. Cover tightly with aluminum foil.
3. Bake in the preheated oven until no longer pink in the center, about 45 minutes. An instant-read thermometer inserted into the center should read at least 165 degrees F (74 degrees C).

Turkey Spinach Patties

Ingredients:

- 1 pound ground turkey
- 1 cup baby spinach, chopped
- 4 garlic cloves, minced
- ½ teaspoon dried basil
- 1 shallot, chopped
- 1 egg yolk
- Salt and pepper for taste

Directions

1. Mix the turkey with the spinach, garlic, basil, shallot and egg yolk in a bowl.Add salt and pepper to taste and mix well.
2. Form 6 patties and place them aside.

3. Heat a grill pan over medium flame and place the patties on the grill.
4. Cook on each side for 4-5 minutes until browned.
5. Serve the turkey patties warm.

Grilled Turkey Kabobs

Ingredients

- 1/3 cup chili sauce
- 2 tablespoons lemon juice
- 1 tablespoon sugar
- 2 bay leaves
- 1 pound turkey breast tenderloins, cut into 1/2-inch cubes
- 2 medium zucchini, cut into 1/2 inch slices
- 2 small green peppers, cut into 1 1/2 inch squares
- 2 small onions, quartered
- 8 medium fresh mushrooms
- 8 cherry tomatoes
- 1 tablespoon canola oil

Directions

1. In a bowl, combine the chili sauce, lemon juice, sugar and bay leaves; mix well. Pour 1/4 cup marinade into a large resealable plastic bag; add the turkey. Seal bag and turn to coat; refrigerate for at least 2 hours or overnight. Cover and refrigerate remaining marinade.
2. Coat grill rack with nonstick cooking spray before starting the grill. Drain and discard marinade. Discard bay leaves from reserved marinade. On eight metal or soaked wooden skewers, alternately thread turkey and vegetables. Brush lightly with oil.

3. Grill, uncovered, over medium-hot heat for 3-4 minutes on each side or until juices run clear, basting frequently with reserved marinade and turning three times.

Spiced Turkey Patties in Tomato Sauce

Ingredients

- 1 can diced tomatoes
- 1 ½ cups chicken stock
- 1 bay leaf
- 2 tablespoons tomato paste
- 2 pounds ground turkey
- 1 carrot, grated
- ½ teaspoon chili powder
- ½ teaspoon cumin powder
- ½ teaspoon dried oregano
- 1 red onion, chopped
- 6 garlic cloves, minced
- 1 teaspoon ground coriander
- Salt and pepper to taste

Directions

1. Combine the tomatoes, stock, bay leaf and tomato paste in a deep dish baking pan.
2. For the patties, mix the turkey, carrot, spices, onion and garlic in a bowl. Add salt and pepper to taste and mix well. Form small patties and place them in the tomato sauce.
3. Cover with aluminum foil and cook in the preheated oven at 350F for 35 minutes.
4. Serve the patties and sauce warm.

Caprese Turkey Burger

Ingredients

- 1 tablespoon balsamic vinegar
- 1 tablespoon extra virgin olive oil
- 4 thick slices tomato
- 1 1/3 pounds lean ground turkey
- 1 tablespoon tomato paste
- ¼ cup chopped fresh basil
- ¼ cup grated Parmesan cheese
- 1 clove garlic, minced
- ¼ teaspoon black pepper
- 4 ounces fresh mozzarella cheese, sliced
- 4 hamburger buns, split

Directions

1. Whisk the balsamic vinegar, oil, salt, and pepper in a small bowl. Pour over tomato slices to marinate.
2. Preheat an outdoor grill for medium-high heat, and lightly oil the grate.
3. Mix ground turkey, tomato paste, basil, Parmesan cheese, garlic, and 1I4 teaspoon pepper in a large bowl. Form beef mixture into 4 equal patties.
4. Cook on the preheated grill until the burgers are cooked to your desired degree of doneness, about 5 minutes per side for well done. An instant-read thermometer inserted into the center should read 160 degrees F (70 degrees C). Top each turkey burger with mozzarella cheese; allow to melt. Serve on hamburger buns with marinated tomato slices

Goat Cheese and Spinach Turkey Burgers

- 1 ½ pounds ground turkey breast

- 1 cup frozen chopped spinach, thawed and drained
- 2 tablespoons goat cheese, crumbled
- 4 hamburger buns, split

Directions

1. Preheat the oven broiler.
2. In a medium bowl, mix ground turkey, spinach, and goat cheese. Form the mixture into 4 patties.
3. Arrange patties on a broiler pan, and place in the center of the preheated oven 15 minutes, or until done.

<u>Spicy Turkey Burgers</u>

Ingredients

- 2 pounds lean ground turkey
- 2 tablespoons minced garlic
- 1 teaspoon minced fresh ginger root
- 2 fresh green chile peppers, diced
- 1 medium red onion, diced
- ½ cup fresh cilantro, finely chopped
- 1 teaspoon salt
- ¼ cup low sodium soy sauce
- 1 tablespoon freshly ground black pepper
- 3 tablespoons paprika
- 1 tablespoon ground dry mustard
- 1 tablespoon ground cumin
- 1 dash Worcestershire sauce
- 4 hamburger buns, split

Directions

1. Preheat the grill for high heat.
2. In a bowl, mix the ground turkey, garlic, ginger, chile peppers, red onion, cilantro, salt, soy sauce, black

pepper, paprika, mustard, cumin, and Worcestershire sauce. Form the mixture into 8 burger patties. Lightly oil the grill grate.

3. Place turkey burgers on the grill, and cook 5 to 10 minutes per side, until well done.

Chapter 12: Fish

Roasted Sea Bass

Ingredients

- 6 sea bass fillets
- 1 chili, chopped
- ½ teaspoon cumin powder
- 2 tablespoons extra virgin olive oil
- 2 tablespoons lemon juice
- 1 rosemary sprig
- 1 pound potatoes, peeled
- Salt and pepper to taste

Directions

1. Season the sea bass with salt and pepper.
2. Combine the chili, cumin powder, oil, lemon juice, rosemary sprig and potatoes in a deep dish baking pan.
3. Place the sea bass on top and seal the pan with aluminum foil.
4. Cook in the preheated oven at 350F for 30 minutes. Serve the dish warm.

Roasted Salmon and Vegetables

Ingredients:

- 4 salmon steaks, ½ inch thick (about 1 ½ lb)
- 2 cups refrigerated new potato wedges with skins (from 20-oz bag)
- 2 small zucchini, quartered lengthwise, then cut into 2-inch pieces
- 1 medium red bell pepper, cut into 2-inch pieces
- 1 tablespoon lemon juice
- 1 tablespoon butter or margarine, melted

- ½ teaspoon salt
- ¼ to ½ teaspoon dried tarragon leaves
- ¼ teaspoon pepper

Directions:

1. Heat oven to 425°F. Place salmon steaks in ungreased 15x10x1-inch pan. Arrange potato wedges, zucchini and bell pepper around salmon.
2. Brush salmon with lemon juice. Brush salmon and vegetables with butter; sprinkle with salt, tarragon and pepper.
3. Bake 25 to 35 minutes or until salmon flakes easily with fork and vegetables are tender.

Grilled Tuna Steaks

Ingredients

- 8 (3 ounce) fillets fresh tuna steaks, 1 inch thick
- ½ cup soy sauce
- 1/3 cup sherry
- ¼ cup Olive oil
- 1 tablespoon fresh lime juice
- 1 clove garlic, minced

Directions

1. Place tuna steaks in a shallow baking dish. In a medium bowl, mix soy sauce, sherry, olive oil, fresh lime juice, and garlic. Pour the soy sauce mixture over the tuna steaks, and turn to coat. Cover, and refrigerate for at least one hour.
2. Preheat grill for high heat. Lightly oil grill grate.

3. Place tuna steaks on grill, and discard remaining marinade. Grill for 3 to 6 minutes per side, or to your preference.

Grilled Lemon Garlic Halibut Steaks

Ingredients

- ¼ cup lemon juice
- 1 tablespoon vegetable oil
- ¼ teaspoon salt
- ¼ teaspoon pepper
- 2 cloves garlic, finely chopped
- 4 halibut or tuna steaks, about 1 inch thick (about 2 pounds)
- ¼ cup chopped fresh parsley
- 1 tablespoon grated lemon peel

Directions

1. Brush grill rack with vegetable oil. Heat coals or gas grill for direct heat. In shallow glass or plastic dish or resealable food-storage plastic bag, mix lemon juice, 1 tablespoon oil, the salt, pepper and garlic. Add fish; turn several times to coat with marinade. Cover dish or seal bag and refrigerate 10 minutes.
2. Remove fish from marinade; reserve marinade. Cover and grill fish 4 to 6 inches from medium heat 10 to 15 minutes, turning once and brushing with marinade, until fish flakes easily with fork. Discard any remaining marinade.
3. Sprinkle fish with parsley and lemon peel.

Lemony Halibut

Instructions

- 6 (6 ounce) fillets halibut
- 3 teaspoons dried dill weed
- 3 teaspoons onion powder
- ¼ teaspoon paprika seasoning
- salt to taste
- 1pinch lemon pepper
- 2 teaspoons dried parsley
- 1 pinch garlic powder
- 2 tablespoons lemon juice

Directions

1. Preheat oven to 375 degrees F (190 degrees C). Cut 6 foil squares, large enough for the size of each fillet. Center fillets on the foil squares and sprinkle each with dill weed, onion powder, paprika, seasoned salt, lemon pepper, parsley and garlic powder.
2. Sprinkle lemon juice over each fillet. Fold foil over fillets to make a pocket. Pleat seams to securely enclose.
3. Place packets on a baking sheet and bake in the preheat oven for 30 minutes.

Green Salmon Burgers

Ingredients

- 4 salmon fillets
- 4 garlic cloves, minced
- 2 tablespoons chopped dill
- 1 tablespoon chopped parsley
- 4 garlic cloves, minced
- 1 tablespoon green curry paste
- Salt and pepper

Directions

1. Place the salmon in a food processor and pulse until well mixed and ground.
2. Add the rest of the ingredients and season with salt and pepper.
3. Form 4 burgers.
4. Heat a grill pan over medium flame. Place the burgers on the grill and cook for 3-4 minutes on each side.
5. Serve the burgers warm with your favorite toppings.

Tilapia Fish Tacos

Ingredients

- 1 cup of corn
- ½ cup diced red onion
- 1 cup peeled, chopped jicama
- ½ cup diced red bell pepper
- 1 cup fresh cilantro leaves
- finely chopped 1 lime, zested and juiced
- 2 tablespoons sour cream
- 2 tablespoons cayenne pepper
- 1 tablespoon ground black pepper
- 2 tablespoons salt
- 6 (4 ounce) fillets tilapia
- 2 tablespoons olive oil
- 12 corn tortillas, warmed

Directions

1. Preheat grill for high heat. In a medium bowl, mix together corn, red onion, jicama, red bell pepper, and cilantro. Stir in lime juice and zest.
2. In a small bowl, combine cayenne pepper, ground black pepper, and salt.
3. Brush each fillet with olive oil, and sprinkle with spices.

4. Arrange fillets on grill grate, and cook for 3 minutes per side. For each fiery fish taco, top two corn tortillas with fish, sour cream, and corn salsa.

Asian Poached Sea Bass

Ingredients

- 4 sea bass fillets
- 1 teaspoon grated ginger
- 2 garlic cloves, sliced
- 1 tablespoon soy sauce
- 1 teaspoon black peppercorns
- 1 teaspoon sesame oil
- 2 cups vegetable stock

Directions

1. Combine the ginger, garlic, soy sauce, peppercorns and sesame oil in a pot, then add the stock also well and bring to a boil.
2. Place the fish in the pot and cover with a lid.
3. Cook for 7-8 minutes then carefully remove the fish and serve.

Rainbow Trout Cooked in Foil

Ingredients

- 2 rainbow trout fillets
- 1 tablespoon olive oil
- 2 teaspoons garlic salt
- 1 teaspoon ground black pepper
- 1 fresh jalapeno pepper
- 1 lemon, sliced

Directions

1. Preheat oven to 400 degrees F (200 degrees C). Rinse fish, and pat dry. Rub fillets with olive oil, and season with garlic salt and black pepper.
2. Place each fillet on a large sheet of aluminum foil. Top with jalapeno slices, and squeeze the juice from the ends of the lemons over the fish. Arrange lemon slices on top of fillets. Carefully seal all edges of the foil to form enclosed packets. Place packets on baking sheet.
3. Bake in preheated oven for 15 to 20 minutes, depending on the size of fish. Fish is done when it flakes easily with a fork.

Chapter 13: Meatless

Lasagna Primavera

Ingredients

- 12 uncooked lasagna noodles
- 3 cups frozen broccoli cuts, thawed and well drained
- 3 large carrots, coarsely shredded (2 cups)
- 2 cups organic diced tomatoes (from 28-oz can), well drained
- 2 medium bell peppers, cut into 1/2-inch pieces
- 1 container (15 oz) ricotta cheese
- ½ cup grated Parmesan cheese
- 1 egg
- 2 containers (10 oz each) refrigerated Alfredo pasta sauce
- 1 package (16 oz) shredded mozzarella cheese (4 cups)

Directions

1. Heat oven to 350°F. Cook and drain noodles as directed on package.
2. Meanwhile, if necessary, cut broccoli florets into bite-size pieces. In large bowl, mix broccoli, carrots, tomatoes and bell peppers. In small bowl, mix ricotta cheese, Parmesan cheese and egg.
3. In ungreased 13x9-inch (3-quart) glass baking dish, spread 2/3 cup Alfredo sauce. Top with 4 noodles. Spread half of the cheese mixture and 2 1/2 cups of the vegetables over noodles. Spoon 2/3 cup sauce in dollops over vegetables. Sprinkle with 1 cup of the mozzarella cheese.
4. Top with 4 noodles; spread with remaining cheese mixture and 2 1/2 cups of vegetables. Spoon 2/3 cup sauce in dollops over vegetables. Sprinkle with 1 cup mozzarella cheese. Top with remaining 4 noodles and the vegetables. Spoon remaining

sauce in dollops over vegetables. Sprinkle with remaining 2 cups mozzarella cheese.

5. Bake uncovered 45 to 60 minutes or until bubbly and hot in center. Let stand 15 minutes before cutting.

Zucchini Spaghetti

Ingredients:

- 6 oz. uncooked spaghetti
- 3 cups chopped zucchini (2 medium)
- 1/3 cup water
- 1 tablespoon tomato paste
- ¼ teaspoon kosher (coarse) salt
- 1/8 teaspoon coarse ground black pepper
- 1 can (15.5 oz) great northern beans, drained, rinsed
- 1 can (14.5 oz) diced tomatoes with basil, garlic and oregano, undrained
- ½ cup crumbled feta cheese (2 oz)

Directions:

1. Cook spaghetti as directed on package, omitting salt and oil; drain.
2. Meanwhile, spray 12-inch skillet with olive oil cooking spray; heat over medium-high heat. Add zucchini; cook 5 minutes, stirring occasionally, until lightly browned. Stir in water, tomato paste, salt, pepper, beans and tomatoes. Cover; simmer 4 minutes or until thoroughly heated.
3. On each of 4 plates, place about 2/3 cup spaghetti. Top each with 1 cup zucchini mixture and 2 tablespoons cheese.

Walnut Parsley Pesto Spaghetti

Ingredients

- 8 oz whole wheat spaghetti
- ½ cup walnuts
- 1 ½ cups parsley
- 3 garlic cloves
- 2 tablespoons lemon juice
- 4 tablespoons extra virgin olive oil
- Salt and pepper for taste

Directions

1. Pour a few cups of water in a large pot. Add salt and bring to a boil.
2. Throw in the spaghetti and cook for 8 minutes until al dente. Drain well.
3. For the pesto, combine the walnuts, parsley, garlic, lemon juice and olive oil.
4. Add salt and pepper to taste and pulse until the pesto is creamy and smooth.
5. Mix the pesto with cooked spaghetti and serve.

Mac & Cheese

Ingredients

- 1 tablespoon vegetable oil
- 1 tablespoon butter
- 1 teaspoon garlic and parsley powder
- 1 teaspoon onion powder
- 1 tablespoon sriracha sauce
- 1 cup low or no sodium chicken bouillon
- ½ cup low fat milk
- 18 oz. box elbow macaroni

- 1 cup Monterey Jack cheese
- ½ cups plain bread crumbs

Directions

1. Place in the bottom of the crockpot: olive oil, butter, garlic powder and parsley, onion powder, sriracha sauce chicken bouillon, and milk
2. Pour in the macaroni and cheese and stir well.
3. Cook 1 ½ hours on low. Thirty minutes before it's done top with the bread crumbs.

<u>Kale Pesto Risotto</u>

Ingredients

- 2 tablespoons extra virgin olive oil
- 1 shallot, chopped
- 1 garlic clove, minced
- 4 kale leaves, chopped
- 1 cup wild rice
- 2 tablespoons pesto sauce
- ¼ cup dry white wine
- 2 cups chicken stock
- Salt and pepper to taste

Directions:

1. Heat the oil in a saucepan and stir in the shallot, garlic, and the kale. Cook for 2 minutes until softened.
2. Stir in the rice and cook for 2 additional minutes then add the pesto sauce, wine and stock, then season with salt and pepper.
3. Cook on low heat for 25-30 minutes until thickened and creamy.
4. Serve the risotto warm.

Chile

Ingredients:

- 2 medium unpeeled white or red potatoes (about 10 oz), cut into 1/2-inch cubes
- 1 medium onion, chopped (1/2 cup)
- 1 small bell pepper (any color), chopped (1/2 cup)
- 1 can (15 oz) chickpeas (garbanzo beans), drained, rinsed
- 1 can (15 oz) kidney beans, drained, rinsed
- 2 cans (14.5 oz each) organic diced tomatoes, undrained
- 1 can (8 oz) organic tomato sauce
- 1 tablespoon chili powder
- 1 teaspoon ground cumin
- 1 medium zucchini, cut into 1/2-inch slices

Directions:

1. In 4-quart Dutch oven, place all ingredients except zucchini; stir well. Heat to boiling over high heat, stirring occasionally; reduce heat. Cover; simmer 10 minutes.
2. Stir in zucchini. Cover; cook 5 to 7 minutes longer, stirring occasionally, until potatoes and zucchini are tender when pierced with fork.

Oven-Roasted Potatoes and Vegetables

Ingredients:

- 2 ½ cups refrigerated new potato wedges (from 1 lb 4-oz bag)
- 1 medium red bell pepper, cut into 1-inch pieces
- 1 small zucchini, cut into 1/2-inch pieces
- 4 oz fresh whole mushrooms, quartered (about 1 cup)
- 2 teaspoons olive oil

- ½ teaspoon dried Italian seasoning
- ¼ teaspoon garlic salt

Directions:

1. Heat oven to 450°F. Spray 15x10x1-inch pan with cooking spray. In large bowl, toss all ingredients to coat. Spread evenly in pan.
2. Bake 15 to 20 minutes, stirring once halfway through baking time, until vegetables are tender and lightly browned.

Roasted Rosemary-Onion Potatoes

Ingredients:

- 4 medium potatoes (1 1/3 pounds)
- 1 small onion, finely chopped (1/4 cup)
- 2 tablespoons olive or vegetable oil
- 2 tablespoons chopped fresh rosemary leaves or 2 teaspoons dried rosemary leaves
- 1 teaspoon chopped fresh thyme leaves or 1/4 teaspoon dried thyme leaves
- ¼ teaspoon salt
- 1/8 teaspoon pepper

Directions:

1. Heat oven to 450°F. Grease jelly roll pan, 15 1/2x10 1/2x1 inch. Cut potatoes into 1-inch chunks.
2. Mix remaining ingredients in large bowl. Add potatoes; toss to coat. Spread potatoes in single layer in pan.
3. Bake uncovered 20 to 25 minutes, turning occasionally, until potatoes are light brown and tender when pierced with fork.

Spiced Eggplant Stew

Ingredients

- 2 tablespoons extra virgin olive oil
- 2 shallots, chopped
- 4 garlic cloves, minced
- 1 carrot, diced 1 parsnip, diced
- 1 turnip, peeled and diced
- 2 large eggplants, cubed
- ½ teaspoon cumin powder
- ¼ teaspoon chili powder
- ¼ teaspoon coriander powder
- 2 cups diced tomatoes
- 1 bay leaf
- 1 cup vegetable stock
- Salt and pepper for taste

Directions

1. Heat the oil in a saucepan and stir in the shallots, garlic, carrot, parsnip and turnip.
2. Add the eggplants as well. Cook for 5 minutes then add the spices, tomatoes, bay leaf and stock, as well as salt and pepper.
3. Cook on low heat for 30 minutes.
4. Serve the stew warm and fresh.

Chapter 14: Desserts

<u>**Creamy Fruit Tarts**</u>

Ingredients:

- 1 cup Bisquick mix
- 2 tablespoons sugar
- 1 tablespoon butter or margarine, softened
- 2 packages (3 ounces each) cream cheese, softened
- ¼ cup sugar or 2 tablespoons of Splenda
- ¼ cup sour cream
- 1 ½ cups assorted sliced fresh fruit or berries
- 1/3 cup apple jelly, melted

Directions:

1. Heat oven to 375°F. Mix Bisquick, 2 tablespoons sugar, the butter and 1 package cream cheese in small bowl until dough forms a ball.
2. Divide dough into 6 parts. Press each part dough on bottom and 3/4 inch up side in each of 6 tart pans, 4 1/4 x 1 inch, or 10-ounce custard cups. Place on cookie sheet.
3. Bake 10 to 12 minutes or until light brown. Cool in pans on wire rack, about 30 minutes. Remove tart shells from pans.
4. Beat remaining package cream cheese, 1/4 cup sugar and the sour cream until smooth. Spoon into tart shells, spreading over bottoms. Top each with about 1/4 cup fruit. Brush with jelly.

<u>**Strawberry and Peach Cream Trifle**</u>

Ingredients

- 2 packages (4-serving size each) vanilla pudding and pie filling mix, (not instant)

- 3 cups milk
- 1 ½ quarts (6 cups) strawberries, sliced
- 1 large fresh peach, peeled and cubed
- ¼ cup sugar or 2 tablespoons of Splenda
- 1 package (16 ounces) frozen pound cake loaf
- ¼ cup peach or strawberry preserves
- ¼ cup amaretto or orange juice
- 1 cup whipping (heavy) cream
- ¼ cup slivered almonds, toasted
- 2 large fresh peaches, peeled and sliced

Directions

1. Make pudding mix as directed on package for pudding, using 3 cups milk. Place plastic wrap directly on top of pudding. Refrigerate at least 2 hours until chilled.
2. Mix strawberries, cubed peach and sugar. Let stand at room temperature 15 minutes.
3. Cut pound cake horizontally in half. Spread preserves over bottom half. Top with top half. Cut into 18 slices. Drizzle with amaretto. Place 9 slices in 3- to 4-quart straight-sided glass bowl. Spoon half of strawberry mixture over cake.
4. Beat whipping cream in chilled small bowl with electric mixer on high speed until stiff. Fold whipped cream into pudding. Spoon half of pudding mixture over strawberries. Repeat layers with remaining cake, strawberry mixture and pudding mixture. Refrigerate at least 2 hours.
5. Just before serving, sprinkle with almonds. Top with sliced peaches.

Vanilla Bean Pudding

Ingredients

- 2 ½ cups
- 2% reduced-fat milk
- 1 vanilla bean, split lengthwise
- ¾ cup sugar or 6 tablespoons Splenda
- 3 tablespoons cornstarch
- 1/ 8 teaspoon salt
- ¼ cup half-and-half
- 2 large egg yolks
- 4 teaspoons butter

Directions

1. Place milk in a medium, heavy saucepan. Scrape seeds from vanilla bean; add seeds and bean to milk. Bring to a boil.
2. Combine sugar, cornstarch, and salt in a large bowl, stirring well. Combine half-and-half and egg yolks, stirring well. Stir egg yolk mixture into sugar mixture. Gradually add half of hot milk to sugar mixture, stirring constantly with a whisk. Return hot milk mixture to pan; bring to a boil. Cook 1 minute, stirring constantly with a whisk. Remove from heat. Add butter, stirring until melted. Remove vanilla bean; discard.
3. Spoon pudding into a bowl. Place bowl in a large ice-filled bowl for 15 minutes or until pudding cools, stirring occasionally. Cover surface of pudding with plastic wrap; chill.

Baked Apples w/ Walnuts & Honey

Ingredients

- 4 medium sized apples
- 1 cup finely chopped walnuts
- 1 tablespoon honey
- 1 egg white

- 1 teaspoon vanilla extract
- zest of a half of lemon
- pinch of salt

Directions

1. Preheat the oven at 350 degrees.
2. Whip the egg white with the salt. the salt to stiff peaks, add the honey and beat until mixed. Fold in lemon zest, vanilla and walnuts.
3. Cut apples in pieces and core them. Lay the apples skin side down on a baking dish and fill the middle with the mixture. Bake for 40-45 minutes until apples are soft and filling crisps on top. Serve immediately.

<u>Apricot Galette</u>

Ingredients

- 1 ½ cups whole wheat flour
- 1 pinch salt
- ¼ teaspoon baking powder
- ½ cup coconut oil, melted
- 2 tablespoons cold water
- 1 ½ pounds apricots, halved
- 3 tablespoons raw honey
- ½ teaspoon cinnamon powder

Directions

1. Mix the flour, salt, baking powder, oil and cold water in a bowl and mix until a dough forms.
2. Transfer the dough on a floured working surface and knead it quickly to form it into a dough.
3. Roll the dough into a thin round sheet, giving it a round shape.
4. Place the apricots in the center of the dough and drizzle with honey.

5. Sprinkle with cinnamon then wrap the edges of the dough over the apricots, leaving the center exposed.
6. Bake in the preheated oven at 350F for 30 minutes.
7. Serve the galette chilled.

Carrot-Pineapple Muffins

Ingredients

- 2 cups almond flour
- 2 whisked eggs
- 1 tablespoon coconut flour
- ½ cup peeled grated carrots
- ¾ cup chopped fresh pineapple
- ¼ cup melted raw honey
- ¼ cup melted coconut oil
- 1 teaspoon cinnamon
- ½ teaspoon baking soda
- ½ teaspoon sea salt
- ¼ teaspoon allspice
- 1/8 teaspoon cloves

Directions

1. Preheat the oven at 350 degrees.
2. In a mixing bowl combine dry ingredients. In another mixing bowl combine wet ingredients. Add wet ingredients to dry And stir until combined.
3. Bake for 40-45 minutes until apples are soft and filling crisps on top. Serve immediately.

Banana Bread

Ingredients

- 2 cups almond flour

- 2 tablespoons coconut flour
- 2 whisked eggs (include yolk)
- 3 mashed ripe bananas
- ¼ cup melted raw honey
- ¼ cup melted coconut oil
- 1 teaspoon vanilla extract
- 1 teaspoon cinnamon
- ¾ teaspoon baking soda
- ½ teaspoon sea salt

Directions

1. Preheat the oven at 350 degrees.
2. In mixing bowl combine dry ingredients (Almond flour, coconut flour, spices, baking soda and sea salt). In another bowl combine wet ingredients (eggs, honey, coconut oil, vanilla extract). Add wet ingredients to dry ingredients and stir until combined. Add mashed bananas and mix together.
3. Place in a greased (non-stick cooking spray 9x5 loaf pan) and bake 40- 45 min depending on oven.

Moroccan Spiced Orange Salad

Ingredients

- 6 oranges, cut into segments
- 1 teaspoon lemon juice
- ¼ teaspoon cinnamon powder
- ¼ teaspoon ground ginger
- 1 teaspoon orange zest
- 2 tablespoons sliced almonds

Directions

1. Combine the orange segments, lemon juice, cinnamon, ginger, orange zest and almonds in a bowl.
2. Serve immediately.

<u>Blackberry Cobbler</u>

Ingredients

- 1 ½ pounds fresh blackberries
- 1 tablespoon lemon juice
- ¼ cup maple syrup
- 1 tablespoon cornstarch
- ¼ teaspoon ground ginger
- 1 cup whole wheat flour
- 1 cup rolled oats
- 2 tablespoons raw honey
- ¼ cup coconut oil, melted

Directions

1. Combine the blackberries, lemon juice, maple syrup, cornstarch and ginger in a deep dish baking pan.
2. For the topping, combine the wheat flour, oats, honey and coconut oil in a bowl and mix well.
3. Spread this mixture over the blackberries and bake in the preheated oven at 350F for 35-40 minutes until the topping is golden brown and crisp.
4. Serve chilled.

Raspberry Tarts

Ingredients

- 1 cup/ 250 ml milk
- ½ vanilla bean, halved lengthwise and seeds scraped
- 3 egg yolks
- ¼ cup/ 55 g sugar
- 2 tablespoons flour
- 1 tablespoon framboise (raspberry liqueur)
- ¼ cup heavy cream
- 1 pound/ 450 g fresh raspberries
- 1 (9-inch/ 23 cm) prepared baked cookie crust

Directions

1. Put the milk in a saucepan. Split the vanilla bean, scraping the seeds into the milk, then drop in the pot. Heat to a simmer, remove from heat, cover, and set to infuse 10 minutes.
2. In bowl using an electric mixer, beat the yolks with the sugar until pale. Beat in the flour. Pull the vanilla bean from the milk and whisk the milk gradually into the egg mixture. Pour back into the saucepan, bring to a boil, and cook 1 minute. Remove from the heat and stir in the framboise. Strain into a bowl, cover with plastic wrap, and set aside to cool. When chilled, whip the cream and gently fold it in.
3. Spread the pastry cream evenly in the base of the prepared cookie crust. Arrange the berries neatly over top.

Grilled Peaches with Yogurt

Ingredients

- 2 large peaches, halved and pitted
- 2 tablespoons raw honey
- ½ teaspoon cinnamon powder
- 1 cup low fat plain yogurt
- ¼ cup sliced almonds

Directions

1. Drizzle the peach halves with honey and sprinkle with cinnamon powder.
2. Heat a grill pan over medium flame and place the peaches on the grill.
3. Cook until browned then place on serving plates.
4. Top with yogurt and almond slices and serve right away.

Chapter 15: Conclusion

I had a lot of goals when I set out to write this book, but the most important of these was to shed light on the Fatty Liver Disease and how to avoid or beat it.

You have one life to live. If you have Fatty Liver Disease, it is not a death sentence, but rather, a wake-up call for you to take better care of yourself. Think of it as a blessing in disguise. You are going to have to make some changes. That's it.

You should ensure that you follow these simple rules of thumb:

- Limit alcoholic beverages and drinks sweetened with fruit sugar (fructose).
- Drink plenty of nonalcoholic beverages, especially water.
- Limit intake sugary products such as desert and candy
- Limit fatty foods and cholesterol foods.
- Exercise regularly and lose weight. Keeping your body at a healthy weight reduces your risk of gout.

I hope you enjoyed this book and found it useful. Now that you have a basic understanding of Fatty Liver Disease and its causes and remedies, I want you to act on what you have learned and BEAT it into your past, where it belongs.

Glossary

Ascites: Ascites is the build- up of fluid in the abdomen that can occur with liver failure,

cirrhosis, and liver cancer.

Cholesterol: Cholesterol is a type of fat found in blood.

Cirrhosis: Cirrhosis is extensive scarring of the liver -- hard scar tissue replaces soft healthy

tissue. Severe scarring of the liver can prevent the liver from working well.

Clinical trial: A clinical trial is a medical research study conducted to find answers to health

questions. Clinical trials are often conducted to evaluate new medications, combinations of

medications, or new ways to use current treatments. Also, clinical trials are conducted to

evaluate new tests, equipment, and procedures for diagnosing and detecting health conditions

and to find vaccines to prevent illnesses.

Computerized tomography (CT) scan: A CT scan is an imaging method that uses x-rays to get

detailed pictures of the body

Diabetes: Diabetes is a condition that occurs when the body cannot use glucose (a type of sugar)

normally.

Edema: Edema is the build- up of fluid in the legs that can occur due to liver failure, cirrhosis,

and liver cancer.

Fibrosis: Fibrosis is the initial scarring of the liver.

Gastroenterologist: A gastroenterologist is a doctor who specializes in the study of digestive

organs including the liver.

Hepatitis: Hepatitis means "inflammation of the liver".

Hepatologist: A hepatologist is a doctor who specializes in the study of the liver.

Jaundice: Jaundice is the yellowing of the skin and white part of the eyes.

Liver: The liver is the second largest organ in your body. It processes what you eat and drink

into energy and nutrients your body can use. The liver also removes harmful substances from

your blood.

Liver biopsy: A liver biopsy is a medical procedure used to remove a small piece of liver tissue

that is studied in the lab to determine the liver's condition.

Liver cancer: Liver cancer is the growth and spread of unhealthy cells in the liver.

Liver failure: Liver failure is the inability of the liver to function and perform its jobs.

Liver function tests: Liver function tests help check the liver's health and detect liver damage.

These blood tests measure the levels of certain proteins and enzymes in the blood. Proteins are

large molecules that make sure the body's organs function properly. Enzymes are protein cells

that help important chemical reactions to occur in the body.

ALT: Alanine transaminase (ALT) is an enzyme mainly found in the liver. The ALT test

measures the level of ALT in the blood. Consistently high levels of ALT can be a sign of

liver swelling or injury.

AST: Aspartate transaminase (AST) is an enzyme found in large amounts in the liver and

other parts of the body. The AST test measures the level of AST in the blood. High levels

of AST can be a sign of liver damage.

Liver transplant: A liver transplant is the process of replacing a sick liver with a donated,

healthy liver.

Nonalcoholic fatty liver disease: Nonalcoholic fatty liver disease (NAFLD) is the build up of

extra fat in liver cells that is not caused by alcohol.

Nonalcoholic steatohepatitis: Nonalcoholic steatohepatitis (NASH) is a severe form of

nonalcoholic fatty liver disease that causes the liver to swell and become damaged.

Steatohepatitis: Steatohepatitis is extra fat build up in the liver (steatosis) and the swelling of the

liver (hepatitis).

Steatosis: Steatosis is the build up of extra fat in the liver.

Triglycerides: Triglycerides are a type of fat found in blood.

Ultrasound: An ultrasound is an imaging technique that uses waves to see inside views of the liver